# Tooth Regrowth

Tooth Regrowth

# Tooth Regrowth

## Natural Methods to Remineralize, Restore and Repair Your Teeth and Gums at Home

## Danielle Ross & Instafo

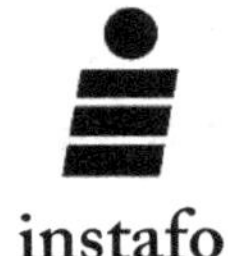

instafo

involvement you take with them, you need to fully understand and abide to their own terms and conditions.

ISBN 978-1-790-53481-4

Printed in the United States of America

First Edition

# Tooth Regrowth

# CONTENTS

# Tooth Regrowth

# <u>Chapter 1</u>:

## Taking Care of Dental Problems

### Vital Asset

Your **smile** is often the first thing people notice when you walk into a room. Happy, healthy teeth and gums along with a sparkling smile can light up any room. But decaying, damaged or yellow teeth are enough to make anyone frown.

More than just the superficiality, your teeth act as a vital ingrained part to your survival. Can you imagine losing the ability to eat because you can't chew? That's why it's paramount to take care of your teeth.

<u>Good news</u>: Restoring your smile and reversing damage to your teeth no longer require expensive trips to the dentist as the sole option. If you're no longer proud of your pearly whites, *remineralizing your teeth* may be the answer.

**Tooth remineralization** helps restore the strength and function of your teeth with the help of calcium and phosphate ions to replace the void left by decaying enamel.

*Sounds a little overly scientific, doesn't it?* But you can remineralize easily at home.

**Remineralizing can help you**

- Grow whiter teeth naturally.

- Fight tooth decay and cavities.

- Promote strong and healthy teeth.

- Reduce the need for costly visits to the dentist.

- Restore your teeth without fillings. *(Seriously? Yes!)*

**Here's an alternative way to think of it:**

Imagine your skin all dry and cracked because of extreme weather. Then you rub on a thick layer of moisturizing lotion. *Ahhh, relief!* That's just like remineralizing your teeth with the natural and effective methods which you will discover later.

## Fair Warning

Before we uncover the hidden secrets to restoring your teeth, we would like to put out a small disclaimer: **don't neglect checkups!**

As revolutionary as tooth remineralization may be, it is still considered to be in its early stages with science even though there have already been extensive studies backing the validity of it.

This does <u>NOT</u> excuse anybody from seeing their dentist. To maintain good oral hygiene, use the information contained within here in addition to continuing your regular dental visits.

With that said, let's jump into some exciting methods to restore and rejuvenate your teeth.

# Chapter 2:

## Start Stimulating the Process

### Medicinal Plant Approach

First of all, have you ever heard of the "comfrey plant" (*symphytum officinale*)? This plant has been known for thousands of years across Europe and Asia, but it was only during the last couple of hundred years that it has gained more notoriety for its medicinal usage.

The comfrey plant's roots are widely used in herbal medicine for promoting healthy bones, healing sprains, improving bruises and other ailments.

*But, guess what?* The comfrey root is also great for remineralizing your teeth according to holistic doctor Michelle Honda, Ph.D., who promotes the use of comfrey roots for gum disease and bleeding gums.

## The Comfrey Roots Method

1. Wash your comfrey roots thoroughly just as you would with any vegetables or fruits to remove dirt or bacteria.

2. Boil the roots for about <u>10</u> to <u>15 minutes</u>.

3. Strain the roots then *dice* or *mash* them.

4. Toss the roots into the blender with some water and blend until everything is liquified.

5. Swish the liquid in your mouth for up to <u>20 minutes</u> then spit it out. *(Comfrey roots are typically not meant for*

*internal consumption due to potential liver problems they may cause for some people.)*

6. Rinse your mouth with water to remove the residue.

Yes, <u>20 minutes</u> is a long time to swish. And let's be honest: natural herbs don't necessarily taste the best. But once you start seeing the results, you'll be glad you did it.

Think of your teeth as bricks and the comfrey root liquid like the cement that a bricklayer uses to construct a building. The solution will help keep your teeth strong and firm inside your mouth. You wouldn't want a building to collapse from using a substandard cement, would you?

Just the same, you don't want your teeth to fall out either. Comfrey roots are the key to having stronger teeth.

## Herbalism Action Plan

Your assignment now would be to try out this comfrey root method.

- Visit your local herbalist or shop online (you can even go on Amazon.com) for fresh or dried comfrey. Buy a few pounds to save yourself from having to make frequent purchases.

- Follow the six simple steps that we discussed prior.

- Keep the rest of the liquid refrigerated, and use it every day for about a week.

# Chapter 3:

## Restoring the Natural Health to Teeth

### Ancient Medicinal System

If your pearly whites are neither pearly nor white, you can whiten them the natural way. *How?*

**Ayurvedic medicine** is regarded as the *world's oldest natural healing system* which originated thousands of years ago in India. Ayurvedic medicine's approach to good health focuses on healthy living through mind, body and spirit.

You can promote the health and whitening of your teeth through the Ayurvedic method of **"oil pulling."**

*How do you perform it?* It's as simple as swishing coconut oil, olive oil or sesame oil. Some people do it just once a week, while others swish daily. Or, every time you brush your teeth, you can swish first. Who knows, you may even decide to replace your old-fashioned minty mouthwash with the oil pulling method.

*And that's not all.* Dentist and sleep specialist Dr. Mark Burhenne recommends oil pulling for reducing the risk of gum disease and remineralizing your teeth. Once you start oil pulling regularly, you may feel better overall because the oils can help detox your system and improve your health.

Here are some quick pointers regarding oil pulling:

- You can use oil pulling as an entire mouthwash replacement before brushing. So all that burning sensation from your Listerine can be a thing of the past.

- Habitual oil pulling can improve your overall health. If you haven't noticed, how you maintain your mouth also determines how well your body functions.

- Pick an all-natural organic oil. Coconut oil is the most popular choice, preferably unrefined coconut oil that retains all its natural health benefits. Other oils like olive oil and sesame oil will do just fine also.

- Oil pulling is <u>NOT</u> recommended for children due to risk of mismanaging it that can cause health concerns (such as lipoid pneumonia).

### The Oil Pulling Method

With the help of some raw (solidified) coconut oil, olive oil or sesame oil, do the following every morning before brushing your teeth:

1. Scoop up a large spoonful (tablespoon or teaspoon if you're a beginner) of oil and put it in your mouth.

2. Swish slowly for <u>10</u> to <u>20 minutes</u> to cover your gums, teeth and in between your teeth.

3. When finished, spit the oil into a bag and dispose properly. (<u>Beware</u>: Pouring oil down the sink can cause sewage clogs.)

4. Rinse your mouth with water to remove any excess oil.

5. Brush your teeth as you normally would.

Sounds like an easy path to strengthening and whitening your teeth, doesn't it? Yes, just like with the comfrey root rinse, the oil may be an acquired taste. But the beauty is in the results.

## Ayurveda Action Plan

Give oil pulling a try, and after a while you should notice whiter teeth and a healthy smile you can be proud of.

- Buy some raw coconut oil, olive oil or sesame seed oil in the store or online. Organic oil is recommended because hazardous residues like arsenic, lead or mercury may be found in some imported brands of oil.

- Train yourself to swish the oil inside your mouth, slowly for <u>10</u> to <u>20 minutes</u>. Now you can choose to do whatever to pass the time, but just don't swallow the oil because of all the impurities that will be flushed out between your teeth, gums and tongue during the swishing process.

Remember the skin moisturizer example we mentioned earlier? Oil pulling is the same idea.

Once you reap the benefits of some of these tooth remineralization methods, you will realize that having healthy teeth is not that difficult or expensive after all. *(Shhhh, don't tell your dentist!)*

# <u>Chapter 4:</u>

# Upgrading to the Superior Toothpaste

### Better Than Fluoride

Let's have a frank discussion about the "F" word...we're talking about *fluoride*. For decades, we've been bombarded with advice about using fluoride toothpaste, fluoride mouthwash and even drinking fluoridated water. Sure, fluoride has its dental health benefits.

But would you believe there's something *far better* out there? You need to give "hydroxyapatite toothpaste" a try.

**Hydroxyapatite** is a natural calcium phosphate compound that's found on our teeth. But it can also be manufactured. You know that old saying about how you don't have to be a rocket scientist to figure something out? Well, in this case, it *did* take a rocket scientist.

According to www.oralscience.com, back in the 1970s, American astronauts returned from space travel with weakened teeth and bones because they spent time in a gravity-free environment. So the smart people at NASA had to come up with a solution to this problem. They developed a synthetic form of hydroxyapatite to help restore tooth and bone loss for astronauts. *Pretty cool, huh?*

If it's good enough for space travelers, it must be good enough for you and your family, right? But how did this creation evolve from the space agency back in the 1970s to your bathroom medicine cabinet today? We can thank the Japanese for that.

## History Behind the Paste

Here's a little journey through the history of this evolutionary tooth remineralizing product:

**1970:** NASA created the first synthetic form of hydroxyapatite to help restore teeth and bone loss by astronauts following gravity-free environment missions.

**1978:** Japanese company **Sangi Co., Ltd.** acquired the patent from NASA and developed an enamel-restorative toothpaste using the same substance as the tooth structure (hydroxyapatite).

**1980:** Sangi launched the world's first enamel-restorative toothpaste in Japan.

**1985:** Studies from Tokyo Medical and Dental University and Asahi University showed that medical hydroxyapatite significantly lowered the incidence of new tooth decay in previously and newly erupted teeth. In the three-year study, the reduction was as high as 36 to 56 percent.

**1993:** The Japanese government approved Sangi's proprietary medical hydroxyapatite as an active anti-decay agent.

**2003:** Sangi increased the enamel-restorative capabilities of medical hydroxyapatite, making it more effective at penetrating below the surface of the tooth enamel.

**2013:** Over the last 35 years, Sangi sold 100 million medical hydroxyapatite toothpastes.

**Nano medical hydroxyapatite** became the gold standard in Japan to fight cavities, and the rest of the world is slowly taking notice.

If you still aren't convinced, then we have some more reading material for you. You can't argue with science. These studies explain how hydroxyapatite toothpaste stacks up against mainstream fluoride toothpaste:

www.ncbi.nlm.nih.gov/pmc/articles/PMC4252862/

www.ncbi.nlm.nih.gov/pmc/articles/PMC3636833/

www.ncbi.nlm.nih.gov/pmc/articles/PMC2908039/

Sangi's toothpaste provides the following benefits:

- Protection against tooth decay
- Whiter and glossier teeth
- Smoother tooth enamel
- Greater resistance to ugly plaque and stains
- Relief from hypersensitive teeth

You don't have to live in the Land of the Rising Sun to get your hands on these tooth-healthy products. Starting in the

2000s, Sangi's product line began spreading into western markets because of the positive customer experience backed by science.

## Different Options for Different Needs

<u>Pre-note</u>: We are not in any way a part of or related to Sangi. We simply believe that what they offer can revolutionize how we take care of our teeth.

Sangi makes products for almost everyone, including infants, young children, smokers, people with sensitive teeth or gingivitis, senior citizens and more. And you don't have to have any problems with your teeth to take advantage of these items. If you're one of the lucky ones who already has a healthy mouth, you can help maintain your teeth and gums with Sangi's products.

Most of them come with a mild mint flavor. Some are low foaming and others non-foaming, depending on the maturity of your teeth, whether you have gum disease or your personal preference.

Prices vary from one item to another, but generally they range from about $9 for children's items to around $50 for the more specialized toothpastes. You may be thinking, *"Who the heck would pay $50 dollars just for toothpaste?"* But the money you spend now can help you save hundreds more in the future by avoiding the need for complicated and painful dental procedures.

For example, professionally whitening your teeth can sometimes cost between $200 and $500. And if you need more serious dental work to correct crooked or decaying teeth, or gum disease, you could be in for a bill of $1,500 or much more depending on your specific situation. That dental work may improve your smile, but you won't be smiling when it's time to pay the bill.

Spending a few extra bucks for hydroxyapatite toothpaste or related items is a worthwhile expense to save you much more in the future.

## List of popular products:

- <u>Apagard M-Plus</u>, which is the regular remineralizing toothpaste. This is a good one to start with if you aren't sure which one to buy.

- <u>Apagard Premio</u>, which is for greater whitening and prevention of tooth decay. This is the one for you if you really want a dazzling white smile. This toothpaste also has a double mint flavor.

- <u>Apagard Royal</u>, which includes a stronger formula for additional remineralizing results. This is the advanced higher-tier one but also the priciest.

- <u>Apagard Smokin</u> for smokers, which helps protect against nicotine and other stains. This toothpaste is also a great option if you're a coffee or red wine drinker. Don't let the morning cup of joe or evening glass of merlot ruin your smile.

- <u>Apagard Apa-Kids</u>, which was the first hydroxyapatite remineralizing toothpaste for children. It features minimal foam for easy brushing, and a yummy soda-pop flavor that kids will love. Encouraging good dental habits at a young age will ensure a happier and healthier future for your little ones.

- <u>Apagard Apa-Kids Gel</u>, which is ideal for teething infants. The gel also features a soda-pop flavor.

The company also makes the following specialized brands for specific needs:

- <u>Apadent</u> and <u>Apadent Sensitive</u>, for people with gingivitis and sensitive teeth. You can choose between the mild mint flavor or the pleasing Japanese citrus mint flavor.

- <u>Denta Apato</u> for anti-tooth decay and restorative whitening.

- <u>Denta Apato M</u> and <u>Denta Apato Premium</u>, which include low foaming, non-foaming type and a mild mint flavor for those who need a gentler flavor.

## Remineralizing Toothpaste Usage

By now you're probably ready to jump online and buy one of these amazing products. *But how do you use them?*

If you already know how to brush your teeth then you know exactly what to do. You should use these specialized toothpastes exactly the same way that you use regular toothpaste, but of course the benefits will be much greater once you've upgraded your toothpaste from fluoride to hydroxyapatite.

Just squeeze a little toothpaste onto your brush and brush your teeth for up to two minutes. It's best to brush two to three times per day, preferably after eating. When you're brushing your teeth, avoid the common mistake of brushing too hard which can lead to gum recession *(more on gum health later)*. Just a gentle up-and-down stroke at a 45-degree angle is all you need to do.

Generally, when people start using an innovative new product, they are excited to see instant results. With these specialized tooth products, you may notice results anywhere from within one week to several weeks. Every mouth is different, so it all depends on your specific dental needs or issues.

## Where to Buy

As we mentioned above, there's no need to travel to Japan to purchase hydroxyapatite toothpaste. Sangi products are as close as your nearest computer or smartphone. Your best options are Amazon.com or eBay.com. Just search for the "Apagard" brand name, or type in one of the specific product names mentioned above.

**There are other products with similar benefits.**

While Sangi is the world leader and innovator when it comes to this type of toothpaste, there are plenty of other products out there that you may want to consider. Similar tooth-healing products include:

- Pearlie White Active Remineralization Toothpaste
- Uncle Harry's Remineralization Kit for Tooth Enamel
- Sunshine Remineralization Gel

You can also search for these on Amazon and eBay. Remember, we are not necessarily endorsing them but are just giving you ideas of what is available out there.

Overall, these remineralization products work like taking vitamin supplements. We take vitamins to help compensate for something that our body lacks. Supplements help bring your body what it needs.

In a perfect world, we would all eat exactly the right amount of healthy food each day, and our bodies would have the necessary nutrients all the time. But in case you haven't already noticed, this is not a perfect world. That's why we need these products.

## Toothpaste Action Plan

Are you ready to take action? Now is the time to give your old, inferior fluoride toothpaste the old heave-ho and update to something better. Nano hydroxyapatite toothpaste is superior, so there's no reason not to make the switch today.

Here is your six-step action plan:

1. **Visit** www.sangi-co.com. (Note that this is a Japanese website, so you will either need to select the

English version, or you can use the handy Google Translate add-on extension in your browser to have the site automatically translated into English for you).

**2. Read all about the different products offered.**

**3. Go to Amazon or eBay and take a look at the various products** under the brand name "Apagard" and decide which ones would be best for your specific dental needs. Keep in mind that they are more expensive than what you may be accustomed to paying for regular toothpaste. But the benefits are also much greater than what you get from regular toothpaste. And as more people in the western world discover these amazing products and they become more mainstream, it is possible that the prices will come down over time. But you only get one set of teeth (not counting your baby teeth, of course), so isn't it worth the extra cost?

**4. Read the product reviews carefully** so you can make an informed decision on which ones you decide to try.

5. **Start using the products,** and keep notes on when you begin seeing results. Maybe it will be a few days, a few weeks or a month. It all depends on the specific needs of your teeth.

6. **In your notes, document how your teeth feel** after using the product for the first couple of days. Be sure to describe if and when they begin to look whiter, feel strong or other improvements.

# Chapter 5:

# Strengthening Teeth from the Inside Out

## Calcium Intake

Which came first, the chicken or the egg? *Nobody cares!* The more important question is...which one of these is a <u>hidden solution</u> to your dental problems. The answer is right in your refrigerator: the **egg**.

But it isn't the entire egg that has amazing tooth-aiding capabilities. The secret is in the one part of the egg that everybody throws away: the shell. *It's true.* Eggshells are said to be 93 percent pure calcium. This calcium easily can be extracted from the shell and consumed to effectively help remineralize your teeth.

Dr. Justin Philipp from the Centers for Family and Cosmetic Dentistry recommends using eggshells every day, preferably in your smoothie or other drinks. He claims that not only are eggshells rich in calcium, but they also have traces of magnesium and other minerals which can help mineralize and strengthen your teeth and bone structure.

## The Eggshells Method

*Hold your horses!* Before you toss those sharp eggshells into your next beverage *(That would be quite painful to drink!)*, follow these guidelines for properly preparing shells for this purpose of tooth strengthening:

1. Boil two cups of water.

2. Add freshly cracked eggshells to the boiling water and boil for <u>five minutes</u>. (This will kill any existing bacteria on the shells.)

3. Remove the eggshells and let them dry for 20 minutes. Air drying is best. But if you're in a hurry you can put them in the oven for 10 minutes.

4. Make sure to break the dried eggshells into small particles. This will make the next step much easier.

5. Put the small pieces into a coffee grinder or blender and grind until you get a uniform powder. Make sure everything has been reduced to *powder* for easier digestion.

6. Transfer the powder into a container, preferably an airtight one.

7. Add a half-teaspoon of powder into your smoothie or other drink every day for "egg-cellent" teeth.

This is similar to taking a combination calcium and magnesium supplement every day, but you get the added benefit of using something you would have otherwise thrown away, and you won't have to pay for store-bought supplements.

Individual results may vary. But generally, after a few weeks of mixing the eggshell powder with your morning drink, you will start seeing improvements with your teeth.

# **Chapter 6:**

## Reviewing the Remineralization Methods

Now that you've learned the different natural tooth remineralization methods, it's time to review each one by going through a series of exercises. This will help you solidify what you've learned.

And we'll add a few <u>best practices</u> afterward to make sure you have everything you need.

## Exercise 1: Comfrey Root

Go "herb shopping" during the week and buy some comfrey root.

1. Boil the root for about <u>10</u> to <u>15 minutes</u> in order to hydrate it.

2. After boiling and draining the root, put it in your blender for a few minutes. You will get a mildly thick liquid in the end.

3. Put a generous amount of the liquid in your mouth (you can also put some on a toothbrush and brush your teeth with it), and swish the liquid in your mouth for about 20 minutes.

4. When you are done, spit the liquid into the sink or a trash can (do not swallow).

5. Do a final rinse with water.

Repeat this process every day, and use the liquid twice a day as a tooth remineralization natural "serum" (before brushing your teeth) or mix the liquid with your toothpaste and brush your teeth all at once so that you can have the dual cleansing-and-reconstructive effect of the mixture. It doesn't get easier than that.

After the first week, do the following evaluation:

- What are the *first changes* you've started noticing in terms of improved sensitivity of your teeth or gums?

- Do you feel like your teeth are getting whiter?

- Which approach works better: The one where your start by swishing comfrey liquid in your mouth, or the one where you mix the comfrey liquid with your toothpaste?

- If you had to grade each method, which one would get the higher grade and why?

## Exercise 2: Oil Pulling

For the second exercise, we return to the oil pulling method. Coconut oil is the recommended choice compared to the other oils because it smells (and tastes) better than the other oils. You can find a small jar of organic coconut oil for around $5 at a local retail store. However, we recommend that you buy the larger container to save money in cost per quantity.

For the first three weeks, swish with a large spoonful of coconut oil and follow these tips:

- Always think about the end result, which is whiter teeth, healthier gums and fewer cavities. Keeping these positive thoughts in mind will help you get through the 15 minutes of swishing.

- Swish slowly so you do not overwork your jaw and facial muscles. This also will allow the oil to effectively reach in between all your teeth, around your gums and under your tongue.

- Don't think about the taste. Keep your mind occupied with something else as you go about your day.

- Breathe through your nose. By doing so, you reduce the risk of swallowing the oil or accidentally spitting it out.

After making oil pulling a ritual, answer the following questions:

- How long did it take for your teeth to become noticeably whiter?

- How do your gums feel a few days after beginning oil pulling?

- Do you eat food more comfortably now?

## Exercise 3: Hydroxyapatite Toothpaste

Visit Amazon, eBay, or anywhere else online where you can find and order a tube of hydroxyapatite toothpaste. There are various options to choose from depending on your specific dental needs, but "Apagard" from the Japanese company Sangi is the leading-brand as of right now. Replace your usual fluoride toothpaste with the hydroxyapatite toothpaste. Follow your same brushing routine, brushing at least twice a day for two minutes.

Evaluate your results after the first week:

- What do you notice already after seven days of using this specialized toothpaste?

- Do you see any improvement with coffee, tea or wine stains?

- Are your gums still very sensitive?

- Do you feel any improvement when it comes to tooth decay? Do you see any tooth regrowth?

### Exercise 4: Eggshell Supplements

Now we come to the eggshell powder diet.

1. Get four eggshells, after they have been purified through boiling for a few minutes.

2. Air dry or oven dry the shells, then break them into small pieces.

3. Put the small pieces in a coffee grinder or blender until they become a uniform powder

4. Put the powder in an airtight container for storage.

5. Use half a scoop of the powder to mix with your smoothie or morning drink such as fruit juice.

Do the following self-evaluation during the first and second weeks:

- How long did it take for you to see any change with your teeth?

- If you suffer from any decay, did you see your decayed teeth being filled up naturally? If yes, how soon after treatment did it happen?

- How do your teeth feel two weeks after consuming the eggshells? Are your teeth still sensitive to cold and hot foods?

- Overall, are you satisfied with your results? Why?

# Chapter 7:

## Applying Additional Best Practices

### Gums Health

*Don't forget about your gums too.* You can't have happy, healthy teeth without healthy gums because they hold our teeth in place. Thus, weak gums lead to weak teeth placement.

Fortunately, these remineralizing methods will also help improve or prevent common symptoms of gum disease:

- Receding gums
- Bad breath *(Yuck!)*

- Constant bad taste in your mouth *(Double yuck!)*
- Loose teeth from brushing too hard
- Partial dentures that won't stay in place because of fragile gums
- Sharp pain while chewing
- Bleeding gums due to gingivitis
- Teeth sensitive to hot or cold

If you are suffering from *more severe gum disease* (**periodontitis**) where your receding gums are really pulled away from your teeth resulting in loose teeth and weak bones, there is a possibility of rejuvenating your receding gums lines with "hyaluronic acid."

**Hyaluronic acid** is a connective-tissue component found in our body responsible for the holdup of our skin and cells. When applied to your gums, it can provide an added layer to your gums and help aid in the restoration of receding gum lines.

- Hyaluronic acid can be readily obtained over the counter in the form of a topical gel or mouth rinse at your local pharmacy or online under the brand name **"Genigel."**

If you would like to learn more about the fruitful effects that hyaluronic acid has for periodontal treatment, here are two case studies:

www.ncbi.nlm.nih.gov/pmc/articles/PMC3690787/

www.researchgate.net/publication/266626802

However, the surefire way would be surgeries like **"gum graft"** and the latest **"pinhole surgical technique."** Surgical treatments are indeed invasive and should be discussed with your dentist.

## Homemade Toothpaste

Have you ever thought about making homemade toothpaste? Now why would you even want to bother making your very own toothpaste when you can conveniently buy any kind from the store?

Lots of store-bought toothpastes have added undesirable ingredients such as triclosan to prevent bacteria and sodium lauryl sulfate to create foams that can be harmful to some. With homemade toothpaste, you get to control all the best ingredients that go into your toothpaste, thus really keeping it all-natural. Plus, believe it or not, homemade toothpaste can be more cost-effective.

Dr. Josh Axe, a certified doctor of natural medicine and clinical nutritionist, recommends preparing your own natural toothpaste to use as a supplement to your regular toothpaste.

One of the best ingredients is baking soda. Baking soda toothpaste is nothing new *(Arm & Hammer, anybody?)*, but making it yourself at home is a new idea for many people.

**Ingredients:**

- 4 tablespoons of coconut oil
- 2 tablespoons baking soda
- 1 tablespoon of xylitol powder
- 20 drops of cinnamon or clove essential oil
- An empty toothpaste tube (which you can buy online) or a jar with a lid

**Instructions:**

1. Put all ingredients into a medium-sized bowl.

2. Mix everything together. Using a blender is preferable as it will mix all the ingredients more effectively giving you a uniform paste in the end.

3. Store the toothpaste in either the empty toothpaste tube or the jar.

4. Make sure it doesn't dry by adding a little bit of water to it.

Now your toothpaste is ready to be used twice a day. This baking soda toothpaste formula is the same concept as products that polish and embellish your furniture. The toothpaste will work wonders on your teeth and gums by treating them for stains, oversensitivity, bleeding and fragile gums. And it can reduce tooth decay and gum disease which can cause bad breath.

## Nutritious Mouth

Tooth remineralization would not be complete without discussing everyday foods that aid in dental health. Check those nutritional labels carefully when you visit the grocery store.

According to Dr. Marylin. K. Jones, a biological dentist, the principle is simple: eat foods that are rich in calcium and phosphorus. These foods are more likely to help you whiten your teeth. And be sure to eat foods that will help you salivate more and increase the PH in your mouth. This will help combat cavities.

**Here's a list of recommended foods for better oral health:**

- To strengthen and keep your tooth enamel healthy and strong, chose foods rich in calcium and phosphorus, like cheese, salmon, eggs, meat, almonds and leafy greens. You should have listened when your mother told you to eat your veggies!

- To help you whiten your teeth, choose any type of fruits and raw vegetables that are crunchy like carrots, celery, broccoli and cauliflower.

- Drink plenty of water which will help you maintain a reasonable PH rate in your mouth. This will also help you replenish your system from your daily caffeine intake (coffee, tea, etc.) and from sweating during exercise.

- It's best to avoid sodas, too many processed foods and sugary treats like candy. This is the same advice you've probably heard from your dentist even when using traditional fluoride toothpaste.

Follow all of these nutritious recommendations and enjoy the benefits of improved oral hygiene.

# <u>Chapter 8</u>:

## Keeping Healthy Teeth for Life

### Dental Recap

So, how much have <u>YOU</u> learned about tooth remineralization? We have armed you with a new set of knowledge and methods for upgrading your dental health, including:

- Applying the comfrey roots as a mouth rinse or on your toothpaste to revitalize your teeth and gums.

- Using an ancient Ayurvedic method imported from the Eastern part of the world by simply swishing coconut oil in your mouth every day to see great results.

- Brushing with an improved hydroxyapatite-formula toothpaste that will put you on a great path towards a happier and healthier smile.

- Adding calcium from eggshells powder to your diet as another natural way to improve your teeth from the inside out.

We expose our teeth to so many things every day that stain, damage and decay them. With all this information, there's no reason not to start applying it today.

## Dental Revolution

The idea of tooth remineralization has been unknown to the general public until only the last couple of decades or so when it finally started to gain traction.

And the good news is that it will only continue to get more prominent with the relative advancement of science, technology, and information to the point where we, everyday folks, now have a fighting chance of keeping our natural-born smile for life!

Now you know that tooth remineralization is a trusted and reliable method. The sooner you begin doing it, the sooner you will heal and protect your teeth and gums.

And that's truly something to smile about!

# Tooth Regrowth